Polly Pops A Pimple

Written and Illustrated by
Amy Korres

I dedicate this book to my two amazing children, Evangeline and Leonidas.

 May you always be confident in your skin!

Love you, Mom XOXO

ACKNOWLEDGMENTS

I would like to express my gratitude to the many people who saw me through this project. Thank you to all those who provided support, discussed, read, gave input, edited, proofread and helped design this book.

Above all I want to thank my husband, Kosta, and the rest of my family who supported and encouraged me in spite of all the time it took me away from them.

I would like to thank Sandy Hays for helping me in the process of editing. Without her this book would not be this amazing! Thank you Sandy!

Last and not least: To those who have been with me over the course of the years and whose names I have failed to mention. I appreciate all the wonderful people who have touched my life and continue to make it more full, bright and overflowing with lots of love! Thank you!

CONTENTS

PREFACE

Most kids go through hormone changes that result in excess oil, larger pores, and bad skincare choices. One of the most frustrating results of puberty is blemishes and learning how to treat them. Yes, people will say "leave it alone, it will heal." But we've all been there, and behind closed doors, we pop pimples. Why not know how and which ones to pop?

As an adolescent, I was obsessed with my skin and having a clear complexion. I tried everything from bad products to doing my own extractions with awful results. I received my first facial at sixteen years old and it changed my life! I was inspired to become a skin professional, and twenty-six years later, I am returning the favor to all of you. This book will teach you how to make educated decisions for your skin, including skin care products, lifestyle choices and proper ways to treat blemishes. This is a must read to prevent, correct, and heal your skin concerns.

Polly Pops A Pimple

Twelve year old Polly is noticing that her body is going through some changes. She is uncomfortable with a pink bump she finds on her face and wants it to go away!

What Polly doesn't know is that hormones escalate and fluctuate differently in every person. From around ages 10-15 years old, her skin secretes oil more often. These changes in the skin make pimples quite common.

Although there is no set age when puberty begins, skin is usually a major concern for both males and females. Unfortunately, the self-esteem of a teen can often depend on whether he or she has a clear complexion. Therefore, washing your face twice a day with a mild cleanser is important.

Why Do We Break Out?

- Clogged Pores/Improper Cleansing
- Hereditary Genes
- Stress
- Hormones
- Diet
- Hygiene

Clogged Pores: Pores that are full of oils, dead skin or skin care products are the leading cause of breakouts. If any of these are still trapped in your skin, you're not cleansing properly. Check your towel after you dry your face to look for any dirt or makeup that may be left behind. If you see some, wash your face again and find a more efficient cleanser.

If your skin tends to feel dry, rough, and look dull in appearance, then your concern is an over accumulation of dead skin cells. An exfoliant needs to be added to your regime to give you a smooth, brighter complexion. All people shed skin every 21-28 days, therefore a scrub consisting of perfectly round granules is needed to remove excess dead skin cells. Natural scrubs are not recommended because there is a chance the granules could be jagged or rough. Yes, we all tend to think natural is best, but not with exfoliants. Natural can't guarantee perfectly rounded granules. Scrubs with jagged-edged granules can tear the skin or break capillaries.

Cells that are preparing to shed off the skin's surface become less hydrated and look like a deflated balloon due to the lack of moisture. The skin is vulnerable to jagged edges which could pull the skin and tear it, so be careful when you choose an exfoliant.

If you already have a natural exfoliant and want to use it up, add your cleanser with it to act as a buffer. It will have less direct contact with your skin and be less likely to tear the surface.

Dead skin like anything else, wants to survive so it grabs on to living cells and cements itself to the surface. In order to successfully remove surface cells, you need to over hydrate the skin. You can do this by steaming or putting a lukewarm towel on your skin. This will fool the dead skin into grabbing onto the moisture and releasing its hold on the skin's top surface. Just like soaking dried food on a plate helps it come off easier, your skin will now exfoliate easily and the surface will not be traumatized.

Hereditary Genes: If your Mom or Dad has had trouble in the past with his or her skin, then you are more likely to have trouble as well. In this case, be proactive and begin following a good skincare routine before skin problems arise. If breakouts persist, you might need additional help to get your skin on track. Your parent can make an appointment with a dermatologist, skin doctor, to assist in helping control your over or under active oil glands. A dermatologist can prescribe medication to treat your skin. Estheticians, very knowledgeable skin experts, can be another resource to help get your skin healthy. He or she can educate you on how to properly care for your skin and help you establish a good cleansing routine.

Stress: Stress is also a major cause of breakouts. Try to manage your stress levels as well as one can in middle school and high school. Talk to a trusted adult about anything that is causing you excessive stress. Life is full of lessons! Remember, this too shall pass!

Hormones: Surges of estrogen and testosterone cause fluctuations in oil levels which make properly cleaning your skin important for both boys and girls. It is especially important to wash after you exercise in order to regulate trapped oil glands and over secretion. Make sure you keep disposable cleansing pads or a travel size bottle of your cleanser available as an option to help prevent future breakouts when you're on the go.

Diet: Poor diet and impurities in the body can negatively impact your skin. You are what you eat! Sugar, dairy, processed food, sodas and junk food are culprits that lead to pimples. Eating too much processed foods, especially dairy products, can cause your body to purge excess oils and fats into the skin. You need to eat lots of vegetables, fruits, and non-processed food. You also need to drink lots and lots of water. Of course, every teenager loves junk food. Just remember ... Everything in Moderation!

Hygiene: Proper hygiene is crucial. Do not touch or pick your face with dirty hands or dirty nails. You do not want to force dirt and bacteria into your skin, making matters worse. You could end up spreading bacteria everywhere with only one contaminated nail or finger.

Wipe your cell phone off. Your phone radiates heat, which in turn, melts the dirt or makeup into your pores creating breakouts. Use a hands-free device or don't place the phone directly on your cheek-Or, trust me, you'll be sorry!

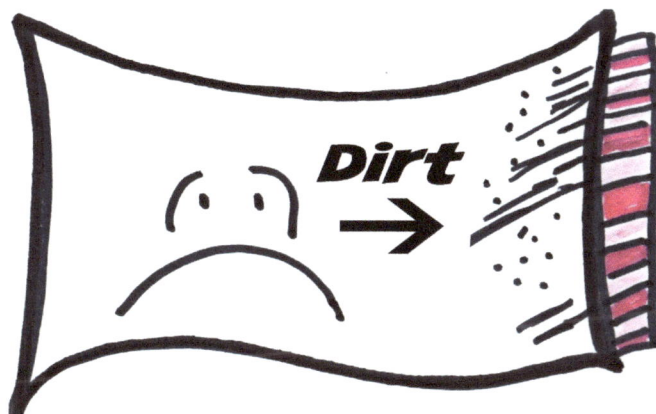

Clean your pillow case. Everyone sheds dead skin cells and secretes oils continuously every day. Imagine how dirty pillowcases can get. You do not want to rub your washed and clean face on a filthy pillow every night. Replace your pillowcases weekly as a preventative measure.

When using conditioner on your hair, wash your face afterward. Conditioners coat the follicle of your hair to make it smooth. When you rinse the conditioner out, it coats your skin causing a breakout. Cleanse your face, neck, and back with your cleanser or acne body wash to remove the residue from the conditioner. You can also purchase a back brush to help reach dead skin accumulation and clogged areas on your back. This will keep your skin clean and healthy.

To Pinch Or Not To Pinch?

Now that Polly has cleansed her skin and exfoliated her dead skin cells, she is ready to prepare for the extraction, or popping, of her pimple. She wants her pimple to go away fast. In order to achieve success and proper healing, she must pinch the pimple correctly.

First, Polly needs to identify which type of blemish is on her face. Many different kinds of pimples can appear on the skin and it can be quite frustrating and confusing for Polly to try and figure out which one she is dealing with. It may be a whitehead, papule, pustule, blackhead, cyst, nodule or milia. All skin irritations need to be identified correctly in order to decide whether to pinch or not to pinch.

Normal skin
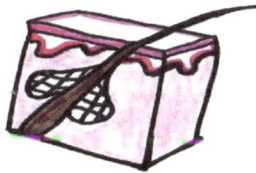

Blackhead
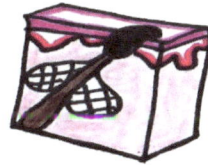

Whitehead
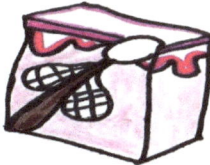

Papule
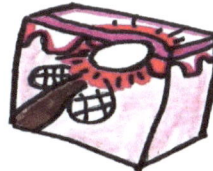

Pustule
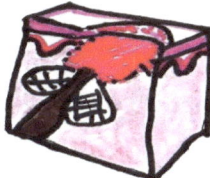

Cyst/Nodule
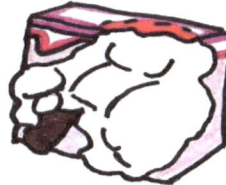

Whitehead: In terms of appearance, they're pretty much exactly what they sound like: small blemishes with whitish 'heads'. These white spots on the skin are, in fact, oil glands. Due to excessive oil production, the glands are clogged with oil and covered by skin. The oil cannot reach the surface and is trapped between the skin layers resulting in the appearance of a white spot.

Papule: If you don't properly care for whiteheads, they will become papules. Papules are the result of bacteria, oil and dead skin cells that are trapped under the skin. Papules are a type of acne that is inflamed and appears as small red dots or bumps on the skin. Papules vary in size from a pinhead to a centimeter. They can be brown, purple, pink or red in color, and can cluster into a papular rash. Papules may open when scratched and become infected and crusty. You should be able to recognize them by their redness and swelling—not to mention, there is no pus. Don't worry if these are sensitive to the touch.

Refrain from picking on papules, because doing so often results in scars. For best results, use salicylic acid or benzoyl peroxide to spot treat the papules. You can also look for products that contain soothing ingredients to calm your skin, such as aloe and chamomile. Since inflammation and irritation are symptoms of a papule, it's best not to apply anything that will dry it out further. The goal is to soothe and calm the area until the medication helps subside it.

Pustule: Similar to papules, but they've got pus—which hopefully makes the name easy to remember! Because they contain whitish- or yellowish-looking pus, they can look similar to bigger, "angrier" whiteheads and may feel painful to the touch. It's tempting to want to squeeze them right away, but it will leave you with a post-breakout scar. Patience is a virtue when it comes to pustules. You should wait until a whitehead is visible and then you can carefully extract it.

Blackhead: If you see tiny blemishes that look like black dots, you've got blackheads. But unlike whiteheads, which are closed, blackheads are open, hence the black appearance—it's what happens when the debris inside the follicle becomes oxidized. Oxidation occurs when dead skin, oil, and bacteria get exposed to the air. The open follicle turns black, giving it the name 'blackhead'. If a blackhead gets infected it may develop into a pustule, so prepare your blemish properly and extract carefully.

Nodule: A nodule is a painful and inflamed bump. It doesn't have pus and is hard to the touch. If your face is full of large, red, inflamed blemishes that seem to last for months, chances are you've got nodules. Pinching these areas is not recommended. In fact, you'll cause more problems because they are too deep. They are similar in appearance to papules but they are larger, raw and sensitive to the touch. They affect deeper layers of the skin. Nodular acne is also often called severe acne or cystic acne.

Cyst: A cyst, similar to a nodule, is a deep, round swollen area of the skin that appears big and is pus-filled. They are formed in the oil gland. Same as with a nodule, refrain from pinching a cyst. Cysts and nodules are indicative of a deeper condition than your average acne and can cause severe and permanent damage to your skin if left untreated. It is important to seek immediate attention from a doctor. They can only be cleared up by proper medical treatment and usually require the strongest medicines you can find at your local drugstore. If topical, over-the-counter treatments aren't clearing these blemishes after a few weeks of use, it's time to see a dermatologist to get a stronger, prescription-strength medicine.

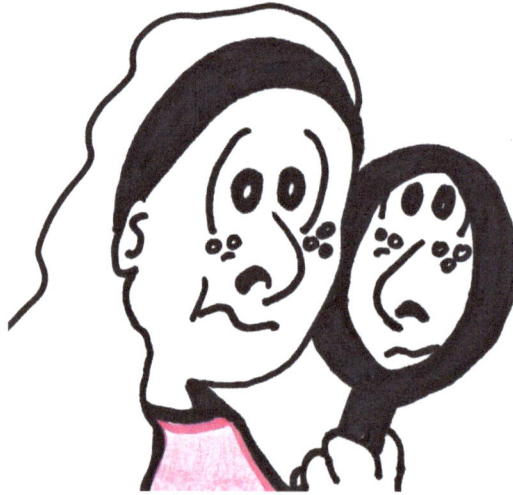

Milia: Hard, white, raised bumps that feel like a little ball under the skin. They are most commonly found around the eyes and the apples of the cheeks, but they can also appear elsewhere. They are caused by dead skin cells that build up in the pore lining because they were unable to shed properly. The safest way to remove these is to get them manually extracted by an esthetician or dermatologist. If you try to do it yourself, you'll probably end up causing a scar, so it's best to put your skin in the hands of a trusted professional.

Milia- small, white, pearl-shaped bumps (Can be mistakened for whiteheads.)

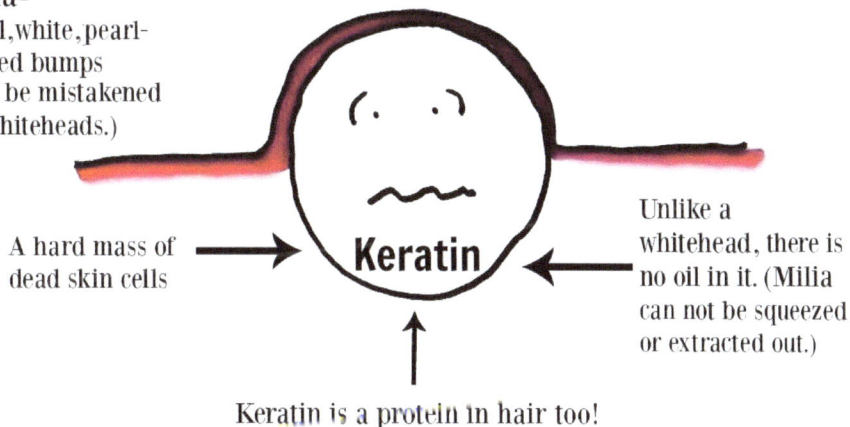

A hard mass of dead skin cells →

Keratin

Unlike a whitehead, there is no oil in it. (Milia can not be squeezed or extracted out.)

Keratin is a protein in hair too!

After the type of blemish has been identified, Polly needs to prepare her skin before she pops her pimple. Oil or bacteria trapped in a pore or under the skin is not in liquid form. Instead, it is closer to a solid. It requires a warm towel compress or steamer to turn it back into a liquid form. Placing heat on the pimple will allow the oil to slide out without traumatizing the follicle/pore opening or tearing the skin. Once washed, exfoliated, and steamed the whitehead, blackhead or pustule is ready to pop.

23

WAIT! One more thing, remember, NO uncovered nails or fingers! Fingers and fingernails carry a lot of dirt and bacteria, therefore they must be covered with a tissue. This prevents you from ripping the skin and getting infections. Tearing the skin can lead to scarring or cause more pimples, so be careful. Also, if you pop a pimple and it is secreting a clear fluid, do not use the same tissue over your whole face! Use a new tissue for every blemish! Otherwise, you could spread bacteria all over the surface of your face resulting in breakouts everywhere!

The Glacier Effect

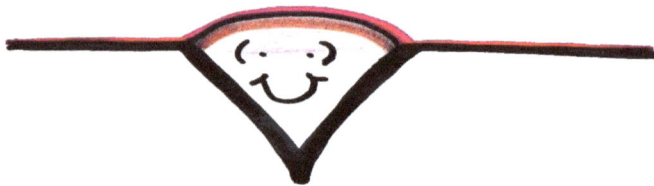

The pinching of the whitehead, blackhead, or pustule is a tricky one because there is much more under the surface than meets the eye. This is called "The Glacier Effect". You will find there is more pus or oil under the surface than you first thought. In order to extract correctly, you must press down, under, and then up. You must keep extracting the pimple until no more pus, only blood comes out, so that you completely flush out the pimple and your skin can heal. By doing this process correctly, the pimple should seal up quickly…like a drawstring purse!

If you leave pus still in a pimple, the pimple will probably come back. To insure you do not leave any lingering bacteria on or under your skin's surface, disinfect your skin with Witch Hazel and then apply a blemish control product. Most blemish control products have benzoyl peroxide or salicylic acid in the ingredients. Test a small area on your face first to check if your skin is sensitive before covering the whole area.

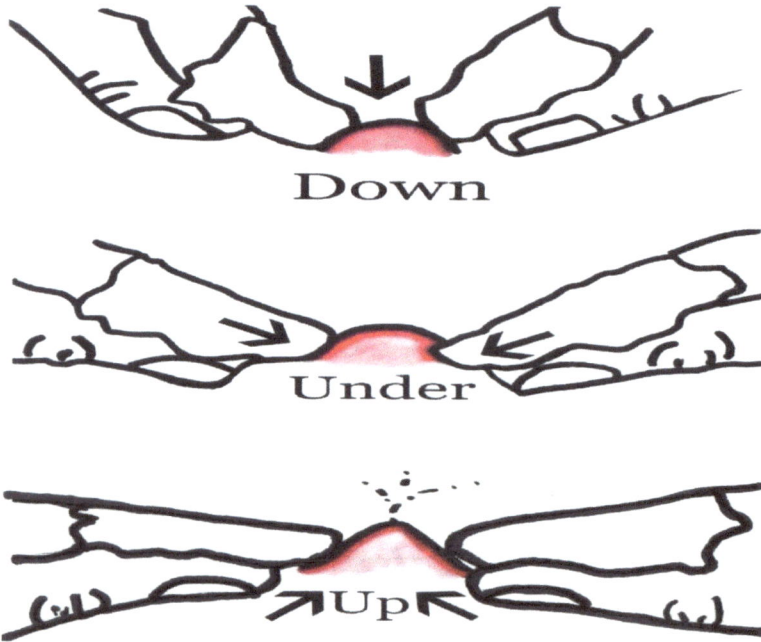

Down

Under

Up

Important!!! A blemish does not always need to be popped. If you can't see the white of its eye leave it alone! When you try to pinch a pimple and only clear fluid comes out, leave it be. The blemish is too deep, and your natural immune system will dissolve it on its own. It normally takes 7-14 days. This may feel like forever in teen minutes! But if you attack it and add in dirt and bacteria, it could last even longer! The only blemishes worth popping are those with pus or blackheads. Both require the same preparation for success. Cleanse, steam and extract with a tissue! Never press too hard on your face. If the pimple won't pop easily, there are other options you can try such as a clay mask or a blemish treatment. Remember! You are not alone and healing takes time.

If you continue to have trouble with your skin see a dermatologist or an esthetician. Either one can educate you on your skin type and answer questions you have concerning your skin.

What not to use on your skin:
- Alcohol
- Bleach
- Uncovered Nails/Fingers
- Needle/Lancet
- Harsh Products/Parabens

The tingling and cooling you feel on your face after applying a strong alcohol-based product is a big **No-No!** The tingling and cooling feeling is telling you that the oils on your face have been stripped away. Your pores are actually yelling, "We need more oil!". This vicious cycle of over producing oil and then removing it causes you to become acne prone. You may not want oil, but your skin needs moisture. Every time you strip away all the moisture, your skin will produce more oil to compensate. This is why using a moisturizer is important in order to help balance the oils in your skin. Once your skin's oils are balanced, the over secretion will subside and a clear complexion will follow. The best thing to avoid this cycle is to use a gentle cleanser and moisturizer everyday.

There are treatment products such as salicylic acid or benzoyl peroxide to help clear blemishes. Use them sparingly and only when you are breaking out.

Salicylic acid helps unclog pores to prevent and correct blemishes. Salicylic acid can also have a calming, anti-inflammatory effect on pimples. It breaks down the 'cement' between cells in clogged pores to help unclog them. Salicylic acid is less irritating than more potent treatments, so it may be a better choice for people with dry skin. It is available in washes, creams, facial scrubs, cleansing cloths, and cleansing pads. It also tends to work well on stubborn blackheads. The percentage of strength can range from .05 to 2 percent in over-the-counter products. For mild acne, .05 to 1 percent is fine, but for stubborn acne look for a product that has a strength of 2 percent.

DO NOT Use Salicylic-Acid Cream If:

You are allergic to any ingredient in salicylic acid. A topical salicylic acid is used to treat acne, dandruff, seborrhea or psoriasis, and to remove corns, calluses, and warts. Salicylic acid can cause a rare, but serious allergic reaction or severe skin irritation.

Contact your doctor right away if you experience any of the following reactions:
- Hives/Swelling or Redness
- Itching/Rash
- Difficulty Breathing
- Feeling Lightheaded
- Swelling of Your Face, Lips, Tongue or Throat

Benzoyl peroxide is an antibacterial agent, killing the bacteria that causes pimples to form. Benzoyl peroxide helps unclog the pores. It also helps stop bacteria from growing and causing acne pimples and cystic lesions. This medication is used to treat mild to moderate acne. Because benzoyl peroxide is so powerful, it helps blemishes go down quickly, but it can also cause dryness and redness, so make sure to use a moisturizer to minimize this side effect.

BEWARE!!! Benzoyl peroxide bleaches towels and clothes. You don't want to ruin your favorites!

You can buy products that contain benzoyl peroxide in the grocery store or pharmacy. It is available in many different forms, including washes, creams, gels, or pre-moistened cloths. Look at the outside packaging to find products that have benzoyl peroxide listed as the active ingredient. Strengths range from 2.5 percent to 10 percent benzoyl peroxide. Start with the lowest strength to see how your skin reacts.

While using a product that contains benzoyl peroxide, call a doctor if you develop:
- Swelling/Redness
- Itching/Rash
- Burning Sensation or a Blister

Salicylic acid can be used together with benzoyl peroxide to fight severe acne. Beware that for some people this combination may be too harsh. It is safest to start with a cleanser that contains benzoyl peroxide to test your skin's tolerance. If no severe redness or irritation, you can use topicals or pads. This combination is designed to speed up cell shedding and clear pores of unwanted oil.

Finally, Polly has popped her pimple. Afterward, she needs to sterilize it with Witch Hazel and a treatment product to help it heal. While her skin is healing she must remember to use a sunblock. I recommend a sunblock of 30 SPF or more. SPF stands for Sun Protection Factor. The rule of thumb is to add a zero to the SPF in order to calculate the length of use before you need to reapply. For example, if it is SPF 15, then you have 150 minutes before you need to reapply. You need a sunblock not only for protection from a burn but also for preventing brown spots where your breakouts are. When you pop a pimple, there is a slight chance you've traumatized a layer of skin. Once the skin is irritated it sheds a layer and the new top layer is exposed and very vulnerable to the sun.

Layers of the skin

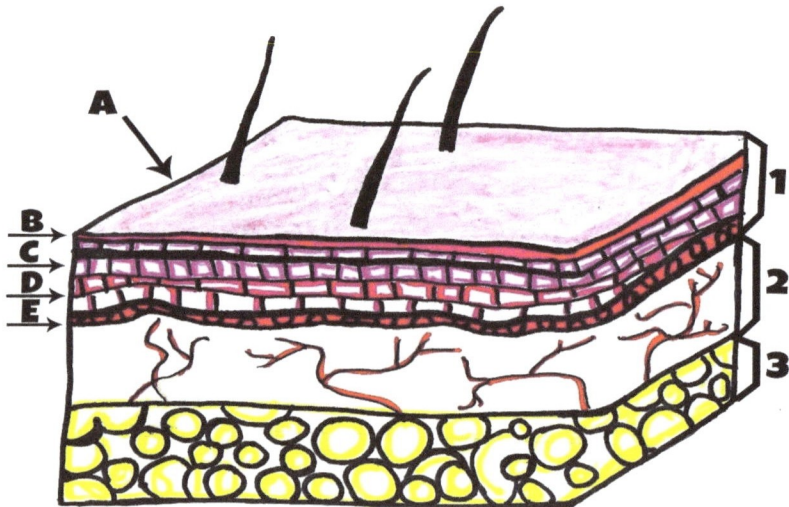

1. Epidermis
2. Dermis
3. Hypodermis

A. Stratum corneum
B. Stratum lucidum
C. Stratum granulosum
D. Stratum spinosum
E. Basal layer

Skin is composed of three primary layers: the epidermis, the dermis, and the hypodermis. The epidermis is the top layer of skin. Within the epidermis, there are five layers. If you irritate one of those five layers with a pimple, that portion of your skin has one less layer. Your skin receives its color from a pigment called melanin. When sun rays hit the surface of your skin, the melanin will rise faster in that particular area turning it darker than the surrounding skin. This creates a permanent brown spot, due to the lacking layer of protection. An SPF sunscreen will protect your new skin and prevent a brown spot from forming.

Always leave a scab on a cut or blemish alone. Its purpose is to cover the growing replacement skin. Picking the scab off may cause more damage because it is still attached to the living skin underneath. Your skin will let go of the scab when it is no longer needed, not necessarily when you want it gone. Be patient with your skin. If you want to encourage it to let go, try to steam it or put a warm towel compress on it. Nothing else!

How To Camouflage A Pimple

Polly wants to hide the apparent redness left from her blemish as her skin continues to heals. Yes, the bacteria is gone but her skin is still traumatized and needs to regenerate to its normal condition. This can take anywhere from a few days to weeks, depending on the severity of the extraction and Polly's immune system. While waiting for her skin to heal, Polly can use a mint-green concealer to neutralize the red in her skin, followed by a shade close to her skin tone to further blend in. She can find concealers at her local department stores or drug stores in the makeup department. She found it near foundations, concealers, and powders in the store. The concealer will be the only green one there. She also makes sure she does not over apply powder. The area treated is dry and will draw moisture in making it look heavy and overdone!

At last, Polly is happy with the results and will continue to practice a good skincare routine! She cleanses, exfoliates, hydrates, eats well, and uses treatment products when needed.

Remember your skin will continually change so be prepared to adapt your skincare routine as necessary.

Homemade Acne Facials

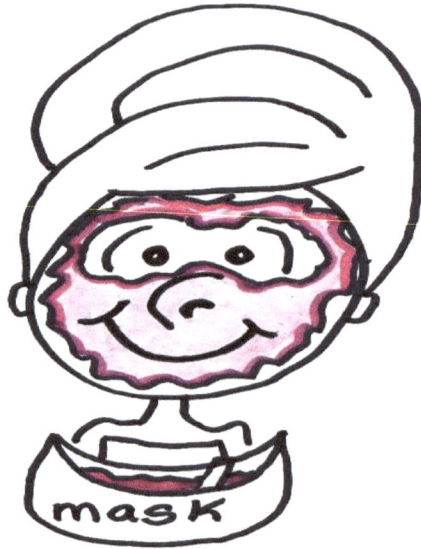

Homemade acne face masks are excellent, natural remedies for getting rid of acne breakouts. These recipes include a variety of ingredients that nourish your skin and help heal acne-related problems.

Honey hydrates your skin and keeps it soft by preserving moisture and promoting skin cell renewal. It is highly beneficial for acne-prone skin because of its antiseptic and antibacterial properties. Its anti-inflammatory nature also helps reduce redness and inflammation caused by acne and pimples. It is best to use raw, organic honey rather than processed honey as the latter may irritate your skin.

Ingredients such as cinnamon, apple cider vinegar, green tea, turmeric, and milk are also useful in reducing acne and acne scars.

Similar to honey, cinnamon kills, or slows the spread of germs, and has anti-inflammatory properties.

The alpha-hydroxyl acids in apple cider vinegar help unclog skin pores and dissolve dead skin cells. In addition, apple cider vinegar treats blemishes, restores the natural pH of your skin, and minimizes the appearance of pores.

Green tea is packed with antioxidants that fight harmful free radicals and help you maintain bright, flawless and younger-looking skin. It too has anti-inflammatory benefits.

Turmeric is good for treating skin problems due to its antibacterial, anti-inflammatory and antioxidant properties. It also helps fade blemishes and acne scars.

Raw milk contains lactic acid that works as a gentle exfoliant and delivers anti-aging benefits.

Apple Cider Vinegar Acne Facial Scrub

1. Apple Cider Vinegar - 1 tsp
2. Cooled Green Tea - 2 tsp
3. Sugar - 4 tsp
4. Honey - 1 tsp

- Mix well in a bowl. Use as an exfoliate.
- For a thicker consistency, add more sugar.
- Spread the mask on your face using a cotton pad and massage it for a few minutes to remove dead skin cells and improve circulation.
- Rinse it off with lukewarm water.
- The granules in the sugar will dissolve quickly and are buffered by the honey causing no irritation to the surface.
- This scrub could be used once a week.

Cinnamon and Honey Acne Mask

1. Cinnamon - 1 tsp
2. Honey - 2 tsp

- Mix together in a bowl. If consistency is too thick, add more honey.
- Spread the mask on your face using a cotton pad and massage it for a few minutes to remove dead skin cells and improve circulation.
- Leave this mask on for 5 minutes or until dry.
- Rinse it off with lukewarm water and apply a toner. If you do not have a toner, use lemon juice, Witch Hazel or a mixture of one part apple cider vinegar with two parts distilled water.
- This is a gentle mask that you could use daily if desired.

Turmeric, Milk, and Honey Mask for Acne

1. Turmeric - 1 tsp
2. Honey - 1 tsp
3. Milk - 1 1/2 tsp

- Mix ingredients to make a thick paste.
- Apply the mask to your face and neck using a makeup brush or cotton pad (you don't want to stain your nails and fingers yellow!).
- Leave this mask on for 5 minutes or until dry. Rinse it off with lukewarm water.
- If it leaves a yellowish tinge on your skin, soak a cotton pad in milk and rub it on the stained areas.
- Use this mask two to three days a week.

Disclaimer

The information in this book is designed to educate adolescents how to correctly treat and heal blemishes. This book is not meant to be used, nor should it be used, to diagnose or treat any medical condition. For diagnosis or treatment of any medical problem, consult your physician. The publisher and author are not responsible for any specific health or allergy needs that may require medical supervision and are not liable for any damages or negative consequences from any treatment, action, application or preparation, to any person reading or following the information in this book.

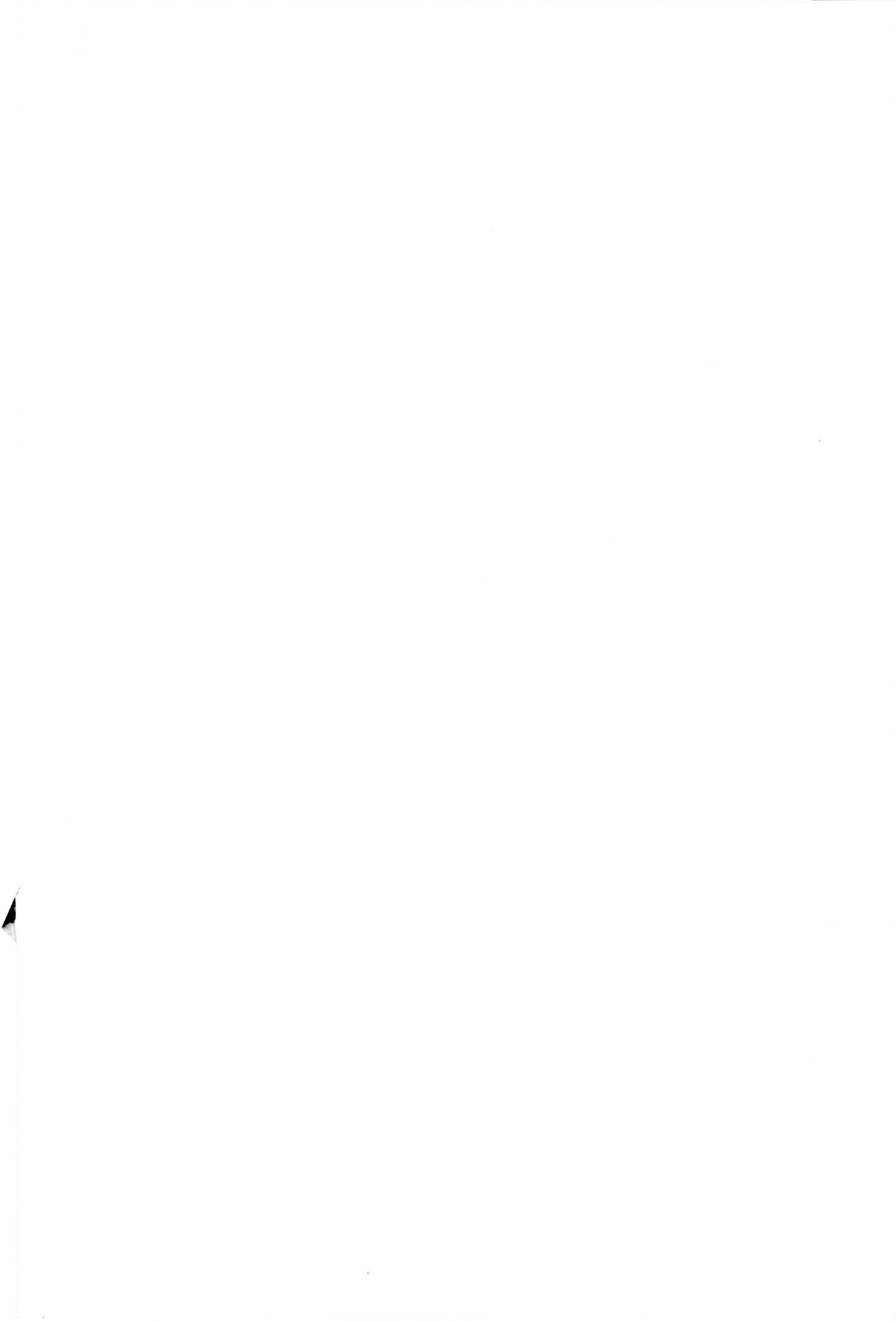

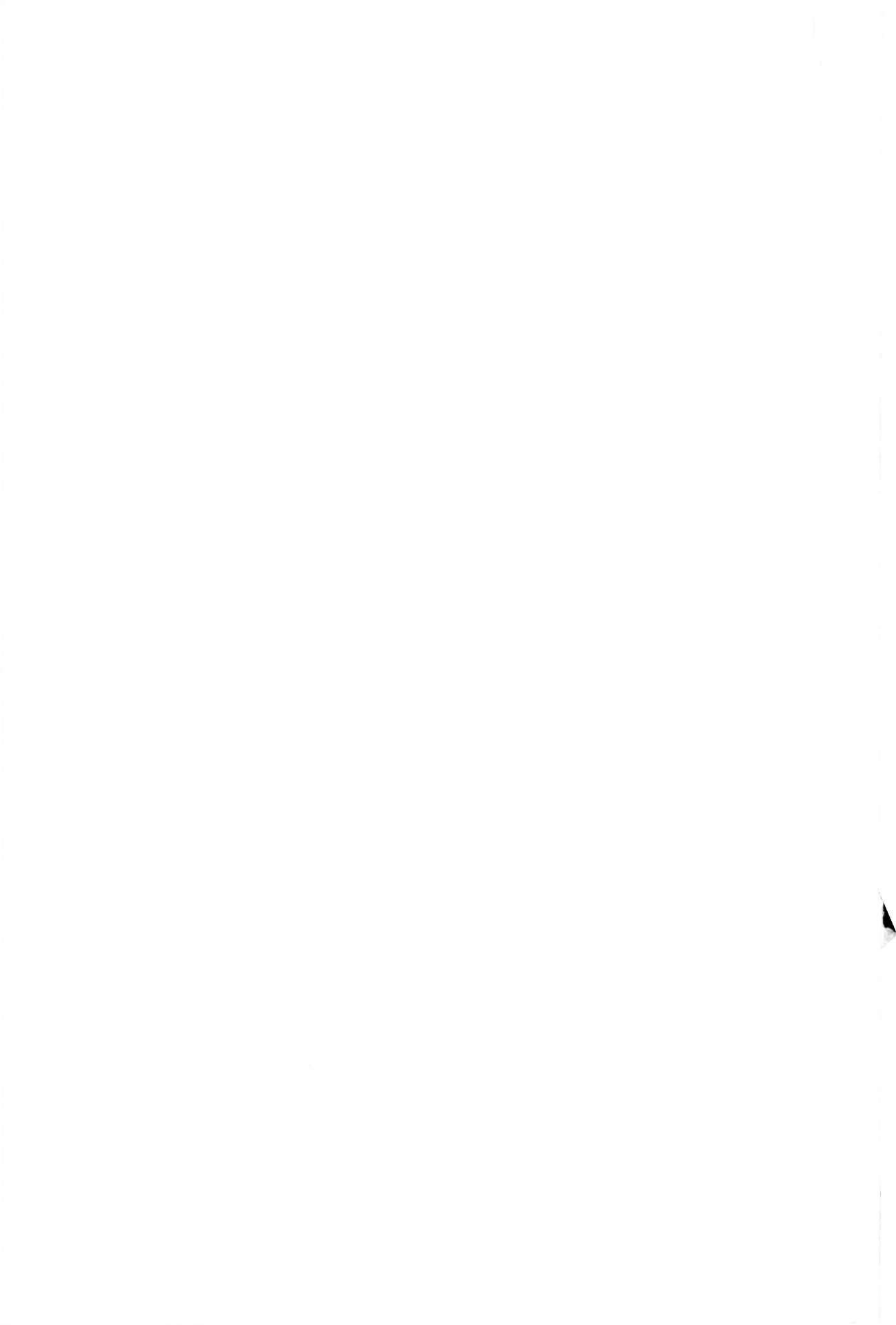

www.ingramcontent.com/pod-product-compliance
Lightning Source LLC
Chambersburg PA
CBHW060832270326
41933CB00002B/59